A Survey of Classical Homeopathy
Theory, Practice and Patient Experiences

Helle Egebjerg Andersen

Published on recommendation by The National Health Service Council for Alternative Medicine
Copenhagen 1999

The survey was financed by The Fund of 1870 (Fonden af 1870) and The Fund of Director E. Danielsen and Wife (Direktør E. Danielsen og Hustrus Fond).

Publication was financed by lotto/pools funds of The Department of Education.

FOREWORD

This report is a shortened version of the thesis 'Classical Homeopathy - and Its Patients', written by stud. pharm. Peter Eldov and stud. pharm. Helle Egebjerg Andersen of the the Pharmaceutical High School of Denmark, with lecturer dr. scient. soc. Laila Launsø acting as adviser. Helle Egebjerg Andersen was responsible for this shortened version of the thesis.

This report is based on a survey of eight classical homeopaths and 345 of their patients.

The survey is retrospective with the limitations this implies. The interesting thing about the survey, however, is that the questionnaire sent out to the patients was based on assumptions of the classical homeopaths regarding the results of their treatment and the developmental course of such results. Therefore, great emphasis was placed on description and comparison of the results expected by the therapists from their treatment with those experienced by the patients.

The National Health Service Council for Alternative Medicine recommended that the results of this survey be published, as it is the first survey of its kind ever carried out in Denmark containing a patient evaluation of the results of classical homeopathic treatment.

National Health Service Council   *Michael von Magnus*
for Alternative Medicine

TABLE OF CONTENTS

THE EXTENSION OF HOMEOPATHY TODAY

The homeopathic principle of treatment was introduced by the German doctor Samuel Hahnemann, who lived between 1755 and 1843. Homeopathy has been practised since Hahnemann's time, but its status and application has been quite variable. Homeopathy's traditions have continued, especially in Germany, England and France. In India it is taught at a number of educational institutions on a par with medical subjects (Bruset, 1995;71)

Today homeopathy is the primary method of alternative treatment in Belgium, France, the Netherlands, Norway and Switzerland, the secondary in Sweden, Germany and Italy (Launsø, 1995).

In 1987, 'Skolen for Klassisk Homøopati' (The School for Classical Homeopathy) was established in Denmark, and the title 'Classical Homeopath MDSKH' reserved for those who complete the course this school offers, or have another comparable education. In Denmark, there is an association called 'Dansk Selskab for Klassisk Homøopati' (Danish Association for Classical Homeopathy), which has seventeen members (Profile of Homoeopathy in Denmark, 1995).

In the past, there have been three homeopathic hospitals in Denmark. They were established in 1874, 1913 and I925 respectively, but all closed within a few years (Pedersen, 1986; 260-261).

In Denmark, only medical doctors and midwives are allowed to give homeopathic treatment in connection with childbirth, and veterinarians are the only ones who may treat animals owned by others homeopathically (Profile of Homoeopathy in Denmark, 1995)

Danish prescription rules require that homeopathic remedies for human use, of potencies up to and including D4 (a dilution of 1:10,000) require prescription (Ministry of Health Proclamation no. 632 of 5 July 1994). All homeopathic injection fluids, as all injection fluids in general, require prescription.

In 1990, several national associations of homeopathic doctors established a committee (ECH) whose purpose is to standardise homeopathic practice in the member countries of the Union. ECH's ultimate goal, moreover, is to introduce homeopathy as a required subject in the training of medical doctors in all countries of the Union (Homoeopathy in Europe, 1994: 24). Furthermore, the activities of ECH deal with cooperation, research and development as regards homeopathy.

It is estimated that 25-40% of practising doctors in EU 'now and then' prescribe a homeopathic remedy, while 6-8% do so regularly (European Committee for Homeopathy, 1994; 8).

There exist in EU-guidelines for the preparation of homeopathic remedies, guidelines that may be compared with the GMP (Good Manufacturing Practice) rules for the preparation of pharmaceutical medicines.

EXAMINATION OF THE EFFECTS OF HOMEOPATHIC REMEDIES

Several meta-analyses have been carried out which arrived at the conclusion that homeopathic remedies have an effect in about two-thirds of the clinical studies made.

In 1991, Kleijnen et al. carried out a meta-analysis of 105 controlled clinical surveys of the effects of homeopathic remedies (Kleijnen et al., 1991), where they, among other things, concluded that the use of homeopathy may be justified on certain indications. In Norway, moreover, a survey was carried out which showed that out of 118 patients that had consulted a homeopath, 91% considered they had been cured or had become better (Christie, 1991). A Swedish survey carried out by 'Alternativmedicinkomitteen' (The Committee for Alternative Medicine), showed that 75% of those questioned reported they had been cured or had become better through homeopathic treatment (Bruset, 1991). Internationally, several meta-analyses have been carried out in basic and clinical research, where it was concluded that homeopathy can have a real effect.

CLASSICAL HOMEOPATHY

In the following a short description of classical homeopathy will be given containing those aspects which are considered necessary for an understanding of the design of this survey.

The word homeopathy (homoeo-pathia) comes from the Greek word 'homoios' (similar) and 'pathos' (disease). In classical homeopathy, one seeks to cure by giving a remedy which if given to healthy persons will provoke the same symptoms the ill person has. The remedy may be prepared through a long series of potentisations, which are dilution processes, where the solution or powder mixture is succussed or triturated between each dilution.

Samuel Hahnemann believed that each individual has a vital force (dynamis) which can be mobilised to fight against disease. According to Hahnemann, the vital force is the life-maintaining force of the individual and is a combination of resistance and homeostatic principles. If the vital force of a person is strong, any symptoms will be strong and brief when exposed to disease, while with a weak vital force the symptoms will be weak and long-lasting.

According to the Greek homeopath Vithoulkas, an individual is made up of a dynamic, electromagnetic vital force and something physical-biological, and can be divided into three planes: the mental-spiritual plane, the emotional plane and the physical plane (see figure 1 and table 1). Each of these planes has a corresponding energy field. Moreover, within each plane there are different sub-levels.

Table 1. Vithoulkas' hierarchical categorisation of symptoms in the three planes. On top the most serious condition, descending into milder conditions.

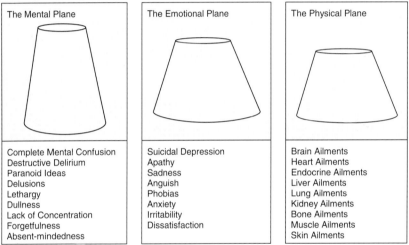

The Mental Plane	The Emotional Plane	The Physical Plane
Complete Mental Confusion	Suicidal Depression	Brain Ailments
Destructive Delirium	Apathy	Heart Ailments
Paranoid Ideas	Sadness	Endocrine Ailments
Delusions	Anguish	Liver Ailments
Lethargy	Phobias	Lung Ailments
Dullness	Anxiety	Kidney Ailments
Lack of Concentration	Irritability	Bone Ailments
Forgetfulness	Dissatisfaction	Muscle Ailments
Absent-mindedness		Skin Ailments

The mental plane is the most important for life, and is therefore protected by the emotional and the physical planes. This Vithoulkas illustrates as three concentric conical envelopes. The inner conical envelope symbolises the mental-spiritual plane, the middle conical envelope the emotional plane and the outer conical envelope the physical plane.

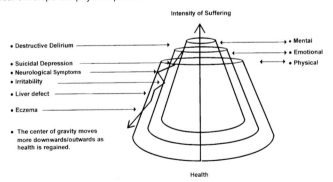

Figure 1. Vithoulkas' cone model with a graphically illustrated curative process.

The vital force is considered to be the force which seeks to maintain a balance on all three planes, and which sets the defence mechanism in motion when an individual becomes ill.

When the vital force gets out of balance, the defence mechanism is activated to restore the balance. In connection with the activation of the defence mechanism, mental, emotional and/or physical symptoms arise.

The vital force gets out of balance when morbific influences from the environment are stronger than the vital force can tolerate.

When the vital force is out of balance, it has the built-in quality of placing the symptoms that arise in a location where they will be least harmful to the organism. This means that the symptoms are put as far out and down on the conical model (figure 1) as possible. Placement of symptoms depends, moreover, on the organism's predisposition, thus, where it is weakest to begin with.

The way by which the vital force activates the defence mechanism is regarded as the best possible for the given state of health and predisposing weaknesses. According to Vithoulkas, this is in agreement with the cybernetic principle which states that control of complex, dynamic systems will be effected in the most suitable and optimal way (Nørlund, 1964).

If the vital force gets out of balance and the defence mechanism is activated, with the accompanying mental, emotional and/or physical symptoms, Vithoulkas considers that the person was susceptible to the given morbific stimulus, and that the stimulus was stronger than the response the vital force could muster. Symptoms that arise are thus considered to be the organism's best possible attempt to re-establish homeostasis after having been subjected to morbific stimuli.

Morbific stimuli that have led to a change in the balance of the vital force are considered dynamic and energy-like whether we are talking about bacteria, or emotional or mental influences.

Cure consists, therefore, in stimulating the vital force on a dynamic level in order to support the defence mechanism in the process it is already engaged in, and which is the organism's best possible response to any given morbific influence.

Evaluation of The Course of Treatment

Hering, a homeopath who lived during Hahnemann's time, propounded a law for how the curative process goes, which was based on his experience. This process is called Hering's Law (Vithoulkas, 1992).
Cure takes place:

‣ from central towards peripheral parts of the body.
‣ from above downwards.
‣ from more to less important organs.
‣ in reverse order of the original appearance of the symptoms.

With his model, Vithoulkas explains why the process of healing follows this pattern. The explanation is based on his understanding of the way the defence mechanism works, and is an extension of Hering's Law.

In the course of the process of cure, the vital force moves the imbalance out to more and more peripheral areas of the organism. This means that defence mechanisms are activated further out and deeper down in the conical model. When treatment progresses in the right direction, the symptoms will therefore manifest themselves on more peripheral levels. The centre of gravity of the symptoms will then move from the mental over the emotional and out onto the physical plane and/or from above downwards, within the above-mentioned hierarchies.

Moreover, this is equivalent to the achievement of an increasingly greater degree of freedom and thus an ever greater level of health, since Vithoulkas considers mental symptoms as more freedom-limiting than emotional and physical symptoms. But the intensity of the symptoms and their hierarchical placement must be taken into account.

When an evaluation is made as to whether a curative process has been initiated, one therefore checks whether the process is following Hering's Law, and whether the centre of gravity of the symptoms of the illness has moved downwards and/or from within outwards on the three conical envelopes of Vithoulkas (figure 1).

In homeopathic treatment one also works with the concept of the homeopathic aggravation, by which is meant that some patients, a short time after taking a remedy, may experience a temporary aggravation. This aggravation is interpreted as a sign that the defence mechanism has reacted.

WHY HOMEOPATHY WAS CHOSEN AND LIMITATIONS

The reason homeopathy was chosen for this survey was that it is a very popular type of therapy in a number of countries, and that in Denmark no patient survey regarding homeopathy had ever been made. Moreover, it was considered interesting to see if an effect of homeopathic remedies could be recognised, as that of normal medicines is explained by the effect of their molecules on receptors, parts of cells and enzymes. In the potentised homeopathic remedies there are no or very few molecules remaining, so that any effect would not be explainable from a pharmacological viewpoint. The survey was limited to looking more closely at *classical* homeopathy as it is found in Denmark. This means that there are no results from the use of homeopathic remedies not selected by a classical homeopath in the survey, and that the effectivity parameters used were chosen on the basis of the effectivity parameters homeopaths consider important in the process of cure. Because of the limited time allotted to a thesis of six month's duration, a retrospective instead of a prospective patient survey was made. This is a weak point since there were a number of conditions we were unable to shed light on. It is therefore important to see the survey as a pilot in which the results are not statistically generalisable.

PURPOSE OF THE SURVEY AND TARGET PUBLIC

The purpose of this survey was to describe classical homeopathic treatment as it is found in Denmark, as well as to give a description of its patients and the results they experienced from their treatment. In addition, the purpose was to compare patients' experiences with the results expected from the treatment by the homeopaths involved.
The target public for this survey was alternative and established therapists, as well as current and potential patients of classical homeopathy who want to know more about this type of treatment. It was also our goal to enable classical homeopaths to use the results of this survey for a critical analysis of their treatment.

An additional goal was that this survey should become a part of the research program which has been running for a number of years at the Institute for Social Pharmacy of the Danish Pharmaceutical High School, in which various alternative therapies and their results have been investigated.

QUESTIONS FORMULATED

▶ What model of health and disease is classical homeopathy based on?
▶ What is the effort involved in classical homeopathic treatment?
▶ What do homeopaths expect from and what are the goals of classical homeopathic treatment?
▶ What factors, according to homeopaths, may influence the results of treatment?
▶ What were the results of the patients who in the respective homeopaths' opinion had attained the desired treatment end? Had such patients any characteristics in common?
▶ What type of patient comes to classical homeopathy, according to sex, age and health problem
▶ What health changes had patients experienced after starting classical homeopathic treatment?
▶ Were the changes experienced by patients in agreement with the results and goals expected by the homeopaths?
▶ Was there any connection between changes experienced by patients and factors the homeopaths considered might affect the results of treatment?

RESEARCH TYPE, DESIGN AND METHOD

The purpose of this survey was to *describe* an object field, and the questions formulated were of the type 'What is?'. This is the basic question used in the **understanding** type of research model, and this is the type of model that was employed. It is through an understanding of the object field as a whole that the formulated questions were answered.
In the survey, a Case Study design was employed, as the classical homeopathic model of the human being in relation to disease and health, as well as the classical homeopathic method of treatment are complex and process-oriented. The Case Study design is characterised by working with several sources in order to understand a phenomenon in its entirety and in its context. The data collection methods used were the Documentation method, in which qualitative research interviews and questionnaires are employed.
The survey was divided into the following three sections:
Section 1   Qualitative Interviews with Classical Homeopaths and Documentation.
Section 2   Qualitative Interviews with Patients of Classical Homeopathy.
Section 3   Questionnaire Evaluation.

Section 1: Qualitative Interviews with Classical Homeopaths And Documentation.

For this section the following questions were formulated:

- What model of health and disease is classical homeopathy based on?
- What is the effort involved in classical homeopathic treatment?
- What do homeopaths expect from and what are the goals of classical homeopathic treatment?
- What factors, according to homeopaths, may influence the results of treatment?

Qualitative interviews were carried out with six of the eight homeopaths. The homeopaths participating in the survey were all teachers at and/or trained by The School for Classical Homeopathy in Denmark (Skolen for Klassisk Homøopati), and worked in accordance with the guidelines established by The Danish Association for Classical Homeopathy (Dansk Selskab for Klassisk Homoopati). They all had clinical experience with classical homeopathy.

CHARACTERISTICS OF CLASSICAL HOMEOPATHIC EXAMINATION AND TREATMENT

The Law of Similars
In accordance with the principle of treatment established by Hahnemann, homeopaths seek to find the individual patient's complex disease pattern, and based on this discover the homeopathic remedy which contains the same disease pattern.

> 'It is precisely this that homeopathy has understood. It has understood that we create our diseases according to a certain pattern. It is just precisely this that is the job for a homeopath to find, because there is normally one remedy which matches that pattern and it is this remedy that can cure. This means also that there are some patients who can have the same symptoms, but who nevertheless require different remedies, based on some single points that differ.'

The Totality
In order for a homeopath to be able to find an individual's complex symptom pattern and find the basic cause which all other symptoms are a consequence of, the total picture of the patient is looked at. This total picture which homeopaths use in looking for the right remedy cannot be reduced to the sum of a series of qualities and characteristics of the individual.

The Symptoms
When homeopaths evaluate to what degree something is a symptom, several aspects are taken into consideration. In order for something to be a symptom, it must be characteristic, striking or singular for the individual. Symptoms are also included if the individual lives in disharmony with his surroundings to an extreme degree. Freedom is also taken into consideration. That which limits freedom is a symptom, as freedom characterises health.

Weighting of Symptoms
In accordance with Hahnemann's and Vithoulkas' teachings, and as a consequence of the model of health and disease of homeopathy, homeopaths focus mostly on mental and emotional symptoms in the choice of the correct remedy. Moreover, it is also on the mental and the emotional planes that people to a higher degree show individuality, and therefore symptoms on these levels are more specific as regards the remedy the individual requires, than symptoms on the physical plane.
In addition, homeopaths seek to find what pattern of susceptibility the individual has and thereby what has been the triggering cause for the disease.
Homeopaths lean variously to the Indian homeopath R. Sankaran's understanding of disease which is that the cause of all symptoms is a basic delusion and that this delusion itself is the illness. On the basis of this model of disease, one looks specifically to find this basic delusion, which is connected with the mental plane, and this is assigned a much higher weight in the choice of the remedy than physical symptoms.

Sleep, sex-life and dreams are listed as some of the parameters of special importance to homeopaths, as these are considered areas one cannot consciously change much, and, therefore, especially reflect the nature of the individual.

Modalities
The complex symptom picture is supplemented by a more detailed investigation of what is special about any individual symptom, what influence different circumstances have on the symptom, and what peculiarity the individual symptom has. These are called modalities.

Essences
The influence of Vithoulkas' essence types on the choice of the correct remedy varies for different homeopaths. One of the homeopaths said that a requirement for giving the correct remedy was that the essence of the remedy should agree with an essence type. Some homeopaths did not mention the essence types in the interview (which, however, does not mean that they do not use them), and one homeopath expressed that the essences may be used as and aid, but that they ought not have a decisive influence on the choice of remedy.

Miasms
Another aid homeopaths use in looking for the right remedy is the miasm doctrine. This can help the homeopath get on the track of the core of the symptom picture. However, it was not all interviewed homeopaths who used the doctrine of the miasms in this way. It was also noted that the doctrine of the miasms can help one pinpoint a certain group of remedies. Moreover, it was said that some remedies may have several miasms. It thus differs how and how much homeopaths use the doctrine of miasms in looking for remedies.

Potency
When the right remedy has been found, the potency must be determined, i.e. the degree of potentisation, also called potency. In the choice of potency, considerations about how sure the homeopath is that the remedy is right, the amount of life force of the patient, the centre of gravity of the pathology, which remedy is being given, and the intensity of the symptoms are included.

> *'If there is something with the psyche and the mental and the emotional, and there is nothing organic and one is very sure about what one is doing, one gives a high potency, but if one is not entirely sure, one should not begin to aim too broadly, then I simply start with a C30 (low potency), and see if it has an effect or not. If I am reasonably sure, I go higher.'*

The Simillimum
Even if the total picture of a patient must resemble the total picture of a homeopathic remedy, it is not necessary that the patient have all the forms of pathology which the remedy concerned contains in order to have the right remedy. This also means that the same remedy can be the correct one for several patients, even though these show different symptom pictures, so long as each individual symptom picture is contained within the remedy.

When homeopaths talk about looking for the simillimum, they speak of finding the right remedy. In this formulation it is understood that to every person there is only one completely correct remedy at any given time. One of the homeopaths said, however, that there may be several correct remedies for the same person at any given time.

Constitutional and Acute Remedies
The search process which has been spoken of hitherto is the process that is necessary for finding what in homeopathy is called the constitutional remedy. The constitutional remedy is that remedy which is considered capable of starting the curative process, which takes hold of the internal imbalance, and which in itself contains the entire disease picture of the individual. But homeopathic remedies can also be used for acute problems, and in such cases the homeopath focuses only on what the acute symptom picture is, and prescribes on this picture alone.

The Case-taking

The case-taking itself, as evidenced in the documentary material, lasts about two hours. The patient talks about his problems and the homeopath asks about what happened before they began. Questions are also asked about the patient's childhood, but most of the time it is the patient himself who speaks. The homeopath starts his observation of the patient from the moment he walks in the door.

Each of the problems the patient mentions is written down and given different emphasis, depending on whether it is limiting to the patient, whether it is something that is mentioned early on during the case-taking, or whether it is mentioned later as something less limiting to the patient. Less emphasis is given to something the homeopath had to ask about to get the patient to talk about it. Thereafter, the homeopath looks for the right remedy by means of reference books and a PC program. In order to find the right remedy, additional questions may be asked.

In follow-up consultations, the homeopath evaluates whether a new remedy is needed or whether a curative process has been initiated.

EXPECTATIONS OF HOMEOPATHS AND THE GOAL OF TREATMENT

Why Homeopaths Believe That Homeopathic Remedies Are Effective.

Homeopaths do not know what really happens when the right remedy has been given, but they assume that the vital force is stimulated or activated on the dynamic plane.

What Happens after the Right Remedy Has Been Given?

After the right remedy has been given, it is thought that the basic disturbance is dissolved or worked upon, whereby bound vital force is released. Thus, it follows that the pathology resulting from the basic disturbance vanishes. Moreover, since there is more vital force available, the organism can now move the pathology to a less harmful location. Likewise, the patient becomes less susceptible to the morbific stimuli he is disposed to, because of the availability of more vital force. But, at the same time, the patient will be more susceptible to more superficial morbific physical stimuli.

The Goal of Treatment

As regards the goal of treatment, homeopaths often work from two viewpoints. Partly from the viewpoint of the patient, where the goal of the treatment is to get rid of the problem or problems he presents with, and partly from the viewpoint of the homeopath, where the goal is to stimulate the organism's self-healing powers so that the whole patient moves closer to the ideal condition of health.

Based on the knowledge of homeopaths of what happens after the right remedy has been given, the following six indicators were used to evaluate whether or not a curative process had been initiated:

1) The centre of gravity of the freedom-limiting pathology moved in the right direction in accordance with Hering's Law and Vithoulkas's hierarchies.

2) The degree of freedom increased.

3) The patient obtained more energy and energy reserves.

4) The problem the patient presented with improved either as regards intensity and/or frequency, or as regards how much the problem limited his freedom.

5) There was a reduction in any consumption of medicines.

6) It was the most recent symptom that changed first.

Re 1). The centre of gravity of the freedom-limiting pathology moved in the right direction in accordance with Hering's Law and Vithoulkas's hierarchies.

Homeopaths consider this as a very important criterion for evaluating whether a curative process has begun. This is the case both when there is an initial improvement firstly on the mental plane, thereafter on the emotional, and lastly on the physical plane; and/or if the improvement moves from above downwards in the individual planes. A curative process is also indicated if there arise new symptoms which indicate that the centre of gravity of the pathology has moved outwards towards the physical plane, or downwards within one of the planes. Moreover, it is regarded as an indicator of a curative process when physical symptoms move from above downwards and from the inside outwards in the body.

Re 2) The degree of freedom increased.
In follow-up consultations, the homeopath assesses, in accordance with the homeopathic model of mental and emotional health, whether the patient:

▸ To a higher degree lives in harmony with himself and his environment.
▸ Is more able to accept himself as he is.
▸ Has become better at creating joy both for others and himself.
▸ Has come into better spirits.
▸ Has become more able to express his feelings.
▸ Lives more in the present and is not stuck in old feelings and attitudes towards the world around him.
▸ Has a better quality of sleep.
▸ Can tolerate larger mental/emotional stresses.
▸ Generally has become more creative as regards thinking new thoughts and thinking about things in new ways.
▸ Is more daring.

How much is focused on these factors during a follow-up varies from patient to patient. It individually depends on which area of life the lack of freedom was found at the start of the treatment. Beyond this one looks at whether or not any mental or emotional symptoms have disappeared or become better as regards intensity and/or frequency.
On the *physical* level one evaluates whether the symptoms have vanished or improved as regards intensity and/or frequency, and whether the symptoms, if they are still present, have become less freedom-limiting to the patient.

Re 3) The patient obtained more energy and energy reserves.
That the patient has obtained more energy and energy reserves is regarded as a natural consequence of the healing process having been set in motion.

Re 4) The problem the patient presented with improved either as regards intensity and/or frequency, or as regards how much the problem limited his freedom.
Since the problem which makes a person seek treatment absorbs his attention and thus limits his freedom, it is important that there should be an improvement in either the symptom itself, or how much time is spent thinking about it.
At the same time, homeopaths point out that it is more important for the healing process to follow Vithoulkas' and Hering's criteria than only happens something with the problem the patient presented with.

Re 5) There was there a reduction of any consumption of medicines.
As a consequence of achieving increased freedom on the three planes, the patient may need less medicines. The less dependent the person is on medicine, the greater freedom he has, and he should preferably get so far with the healing process, that the further use of medicines can be reduced by his own volition.

Re 6) It was the most recent symptom that changed first.
Homeopaths also remarked on this part of Hering's Law, namely that it is indicative of a healing process if the most recently appearing symptoms become better first. On the basis of the interviews as a whole and the documentary material, this point seems, however, to be secondary compared to whether the centre of gravity of the freedom-limiting pathology has moved in the right direction (see point 1 above) and whether the degree of freedom has increased.
This part of Hering's Law includes any suppressed symptoms which might reappear briefly after starting homeopathic treatment.

In a curative process, such symptoms will typically reappear in reverse sequence to the order they were suppressed in. When the symptom that was last suppressed is also the first to briefly return, this indicates a healing process.

However, the latter is not a requirement for the healing process, but the homeopaths said it often happens that old suppressed symptoms return very briefly. The organism or the vital force is attributed a kind of consistency, which in the healing process makes it manifest suppressed symptoms in the reverse order of that they originally appeared in, before vanishing.

Based on the above-mentioned parameters, homeopaths evaluate whether a curative process has been set in motion, and whether the patient thus, as a whole, has come closer to the ideal condition of health, which is the goal of homeopathic treatment.

Nothing needs to happen regarding the above-mentioned parameters in order for the goal of treatment to be achieved, but, as a whole, the patient should have moved closer to the ideal condition of health. This means that no suppression should have occurred, i.e. that the centre of gravity of the pathology moved to a deeper level, according to Hering's and Vithoulkas' criteria.

Paradigm Discussion

Compared with the *subject-oriented paradigm (Launsø 1996)*, where the ideal of therapy consists of a learning process and personal development both for the patient and the therapist, through interpretation of subjective content, the homeopathic ideal of practice as regards the learning and personal development of the patient is the same, but the method is different. Even if homeopaths believe that the conversation between patient and homeopath can start a curative process, it is known, from experience, that it is the homeopathic remedy which indirectly sets the curative process in motion by stimulating and activating the organism's self-healing force, whereby learning and personal development follow.

The scientific ideal of the *mechanistic object paradigm ((Launsø 1996)* is the empirical testing of disease theories as regards causal connections. The same actually applies to homeopathic practice where, however, there is no talk of reductionistic causal relationships. Which causes lead to what effects and which effects may result from what causes, is completely unique for each individual. It is the pattern in these cause-effect relationships which homeopaths seek to unravel in order to find the remedy that stimulates the organism to self-healing. It is evidently not a question of controlling the individual symptom on the basis of a reductionistic model of causal connection.

FACTORS HOMEOPATHS CONSIDER MAY AFFECT THE RESULTS OF TREATMENT

As will be apparent below, the factors that are considered important for the effectiveness of homeopathic treatment are related to both finding the right remedy, as well as the organism's ability to continue any self-healing process that may get started.

In order for homeopaths to be able to find and give the right remedy, it is important that the patient is *open* and *honest*. Beyond this, homeopaths stress that it is important for the patient to have *several consultations*. This is because it may be difficult to find the right remedy, and because it is first on checking whether a healing process has been initiated, that the homeopath can evaluate whether the right remedy was given or not.

There are some patients homeopaths know by experience are difficult to treat. These are, among others, patients who during homeopathic treatment take *hormone preparations,* especially *cortisone*. They believe these medicines to have such a strong regulating effect on the organism, that any initiated homeopathic curative process may be impeded and stopped.

The most difficult patients are those who have a *very weak* vital force available for the healing process. In that connection, the homeopaths noted that children are less difficult to treat than adults, as children have not been exposed to so many morbific influences and therefore usually have an abundant vital force.

As the right remedy is found on the basis of the individual's symptom picture, homeopaths say that it can be difficult to find the right remedy for persons who present with very *few symptoms*.

Beyond this, it is said that conditions which one has tried to resolve by *surgery* are very difficult to cure.

Diet, Lifestyle and Allopathic Medicine

Homeopaths do not always advise their patients as regards diet, lifestyle and the use of medicines, unless extreme circumstances warrant it. The reason for this is that they consider, and have experience to back it up, that when the right remedy has been given, one will no longer feel any need for an extreme lifestyle, and the need for medicines will drop. Homeopaths see these changes as indicators of a curative process set in motion.

The Therapeutic Value of the Case-taking Itself

Even though it is considered that the case-taking itself can start the same process as the right remedy, homeopaths know by experience that the effect of the case-taking does not last as long as giving the right remedy. One homeopath, however, stated that many in-depth consultations might achieve the same effect as the correct remedy and considered the homeopathic curative process as a combination of the remedy and the consultation.

The case-taking is therefore considered capable of setting something in motion, but this mental processing need not be a prerequisite in order to achieve an effect by homeopathic treatment. Support for this is the fact that animals and children also may be cured by means of homeopathic remedies.

CONCLUSIONS

Based on of the homeopathic model of human beings in relation to disease and health, and the curative process evaluation criteria, the very simplified model below was drawn.
The area in the triangle represents the amount of vital force and the degree of freedom. Morbific influences and suppressive treatments move the individual further away from the ideal level of health. The self-healing potential and stimulation of the vital force causes the individual to move closer to the ideal condition of health. Moreover, the symptoms produced are unique for the individual concerned.

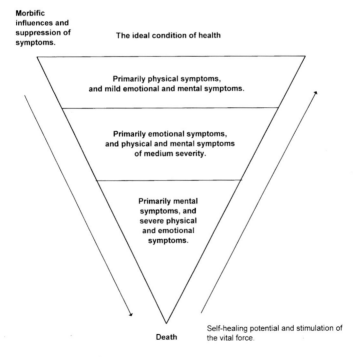

Figure 2. Morbific influences and suppressive treatments move the individual further away from the ideal level of health. The self-healing potential and stimulation of the vital force causes the individual to move closer to the ideal condition of health.

The basic ideas of homeopathy can be summarised briefly as follows:

An individual's disease complex is considered as a unique product of the morbific stimuli the individual is susceptible to and the best possible way for the vital force to react when unable to deal with the morbific influences it is exposed to.
The individual's susceptibility and areas of reaction depend on genetic and miasmatic predispositions, and on what stimuli he has been exposed to in the course of life.
Cure is a question of stimulating the individual's self-healing power through a knowledge of his complex disease pattern.
The possibility of finding the right remedy, and, thus, the possibility of getting a good result from treatment depends on the homeopath's experience, knowledge and intuition, and on the patient's openness and honesty. Moreover, the effect of treatment depends on the patient's vital force and the number of factors that operate against a cure.

Section 2 Qualitative Interviews with Patients of Classical Homeopathy.

In this section the following question will be illuminated:

▶ What were the results of the patients who in the respective homeopaths' opinion had attained the desired treatment end? Had such patients any characteristics in common?

The answer was based on qualitative research interviews. Five patients were interviewed. These patients fulfilled all the criteria of having attained the desired treatment result, as judged by the homeopath concerned. The five patients had completed treatment among three different homeopaths. Each course of treatment will be reviewed briefly, followed by a summary and evaluation in relation to expectations and goals of the homeopaths.

Patient 1: Treatment began about 1991. There were about 10 consultations.
This was a 57-year old woman who came for treatment as she had been suffering from narcolepsy since 1976. Narcolepsy is characterised by the paroxysmal appearance of sleep-like states.
She did not think that the first tablet given was the right one, but after taking the next one, she passed through a short period a week later, lasting a few days, during which she felt very unhappy and depressed. Her consumption of medicine was reduced from a daily dose of 70-80 mg methylphenidal (Ritalin) to 20-25 mg.
Beyond the fact that the problem she came with got better, she had experienced greatly improved spirits, that she was no longer as sad, that her self respect had increased, that she had become better at saying no to others, that she felt stronger and more creative than before (she was playing the piano again, which she had not done for many years). Moreover, she felt more equal with other people and did not allow herself to be stepped on. She felt that she clearly was in greater harmony with her environment and functioned better at her job in relation to earlier. She felt that her general well being definitely had been improved.
She did not experience any great changes as regards sleep quality, but had begun to talk in her sleep when feeling fine, which she had not done earlier. She had, moreover, 'worked' through some of the things that appeared in her dreams.

Patient 2: Treatment began in August 1994. There was one consultation.
This was a 52-year old woman who came for treatment because of cystitis. She had suffered from recurring cystitis since childhood.
A few days after taking two homeopathic tablets she had strong bladder pains. After these pains were gone, the cystitis had vanished.
Beyond the fact that the problem she presented with had disappeared, she had also experienced greater physical well-being and was more able to release suppressed anger. She had become better at tackling conflicts and had dropped some friends, which she felt good about. She felt more relaxed in comparison to before. Further, she felt more creative and was drinking less alcohol.
She experienced the consultation with the homeopath as a therapy in itself, and the conversation with the homeopath helped her to gain a greater spiritual insight, especially about near-death experiences.
It must be mentioned that before consulting a homeopath she had been spiritually oriented.

Patient 3: Treatment began in the Autumn of 1993. There were two consultations.
This was a 69-year old woman whose reasons for seeking treatment were that she had been through several weeks of menstrual bleeding and was suffering from iron deficiency. Moreover, she had been experiencing strong mental stress, as she had lost her parents and her husband, and her son had become strongly neurotic, all within a few years.
The first three days after consulting the homeopath, the bleeding became more profuse, she became more depressed and was generally worse. Thereafter, the bleeding stopped, the iron percentage rose and she experienced a short lasting euphoric state of joy at being alive.
Some time later she had experienced a slight relapse, and was given another homeopathic tablet, whereafter the problem did not reappear.
Beyond the fact that the problem she presented with had vanished, she had also noted that a troublesome brown spot on her cheek, which often gave small sores and eruptions, had disappeared. She could also sleep well again; a tendency to sinusitis was gone; she had started to work again; she had obtained more energy; coffee did not taste good any longer; she had returned to being her real self; she had again a

feeling of contact with the spiritual; and had become more creative. During the depression, she had felt it was almost painful to do the things she used to feel pleasure in doing. This joy had returned. She had also become more conscious about her relations with other people and had obtained more zest for life.

Patient 4: Treatment began in 1993. There were five consultations.
This was a 27-year old woman who came for treatment as she had been suffering from severe acne over the whole body. It had been a problem for about ten years.
After the first consultation, and after taking the homeopathic tablet, the skin problem vanished. She had not had the problem since.
After the skin problem had vanished, she continued consulting the homeopath regularly in order to work on some mental problems, because the remedy she was given for the skin problem also had started a mental process going. After seeing the homeopath for the second time, a strong weeping spell began the day after taking the tablet, lasting for about a week.
Beyond the fact that the primary problem she presented with had disappeared, she had also experienced that she had become more aware of her body and had obtained a greater degree of general well being. She felt more in mental and emotional balance; she had greater self confidence, had become more sure of herself and had become better at concentrating. She felt no longer as restless, and had become more relaxed. She felt, moreover, that she had greater reserves of energy on a daily basis in relation to previously, and no longer had any feelings of always 'being in the wrong place'. Moreover, she was better able to implement her ideas than before, and was no longer as excessively desirous of pleasing others.
At the time of the interview, she felt much happier than previously, and felt 'that she had straightened out her life', which, among other things, had resulted in her finding a new circle of friends.

Patient 5: Treatment began about 1994. There was one consultation.
This was a 24-year old woman who wanted treatment for vomiting during pregnancy, more than she thought could be attributed to her condition. She was afraid that it was due to a mental block present since childhood, which caused loathing for food and nausea. If the block were not removed she was afraid the child would be insufficiently nourished.
After the consultation, a week passed before she got the remedy. During this week nothing had happened with her problem. Three weeks after taking the tablet she had experienced neither vomiting, diarrhoea nor nausea. After a month without problems she had had a bout with diarrhoea and vomiting, but with the exception of diarrhoea one time, had not had these problems since. Beyond the fact that the problems she presented with had disappeared, she no longer had any loathing of food, she no longer felt blocked to the same extent as before, and she felt more present in her dreams. Moreover, her fear of heights and especially her claustrophobia had improved, which was a great release for her. She felt more self-confident and had become better at thinking her problems through and solved them in different ways than before. Previously she would assume responsibility for everything and everyone, which had been a problem for her. Now she had become better at setting aside this compulsion for responsibility, and would only take responsibility for herself, no longer feeling the need to control everything. She felt happier, less worried about the future, and had become better at saying what she was thinking and 'letting things out'. Moreover, her creativity had increased, and she felt that she had become more relaxed. In addition, she had become interested in health food, which she had not been earlier. She had become better at living in the present, and the anxiety which she had suffered much from was almost gone. Furthermore, she felt more serene in her relations with other people.

Summary and Evaluation of the Course of Treatment in Relation to The Results and Goals Expected by the Homeopaths.

The five patients interviewed were women between the ages of 24 to 69 years. They came to the homeopath because of a physical or organic problem. In four out of the five cases, the condition they presented with had completely vanished. In the last case, the frequency of attacks was reduced substantially, resulting in a reduction of the consumption of medicine.
Four of the patients had experienced an aggravation.
The psychological changes several of the patients experienced included: the attainment of greater self-confidence and more courage; doing things they enjoyed more often; seeking to a greater extent to change things they were dissatisfied with; to a greater degree seeking to create joy both for themselves and others; accepting themselves more as they were, and to a greater degree expressing who they really were. They were less worried on a daily basis, had become better at expressing their feelings, and had become more creative, more often finding new ways to solve their problems; they had obtained a better quality of

sleep, were in better spirits, had a greater joy of life, greater daily energy reserves, and had become more serene in their relations with other people.

In relation to the homeopathic evaluation, these patients' experiences after starting homeopathic treatment showed them approaching the ideal condition of health. In relation to the evaluation indicators, they had all obtained greater mental, emotional and physical freedom; they had obtained more energy, and the problem they presented with had disappeared or become better. The consumption of medicine before treatment started had been reduced or stopped entirely, although one of the patients (P5) had not reduced her use of medicines for asthma, but, all in all, she had achieved a greater freedom, as there had occurred many positive psychological changes. With four of the patients, no new problem had arisen, but with one of the patients (P2) there had been a period of anxiety in connection with a trip to South America, which was later resolved by healing.

Since there arose anxiety in this patient after the physical problem had disappeared, was this not a suppression? It is difficult to judge, as there were special external circumstances in this patent's life. But, all in all, she had attained greater freedom, she had experienced several positive changes, and her anxiety was gone.

On the basis of the data at hand, it was not possible to judge to what extent the problem that came last was the one that changed first.

What Characterised the Five Patients Interviewed?

Understanding of Disease

It was characteristic that all patients had a psychosomatic understanding of disease and some of them also a spiritual awareness of disease. Three of the patients had a psychosomatic understanding of their illness before starting homeopathic treatment. P3 said, among other things: *'But then there came a situation in which I received a very strong psychological stress. And this resulted in menstrual bleeding, which lasted for some weeks.'*

With the last two patients, the homeopathic treatment had contributed to an increased awareness of a connection between body and mind, P1 replied the following to a question about whether her understanding of disease and health had changed after receiving homeopathic treatment: *'Yes, it has to a great extent. One thinks of the body in another way. And especially that about treating disease, which in homeopathy is not considered as the ultimate goal. One looks at the human being as a whole. That I think is exciting and when I hear of such a thing, I try to understand it and find out more about it.'*

It is, however, interesting that in all the cases it was a physical problem the patients came to get treatment for, despite an understanding of disease as being psychosomatic.

Understanding of the Homeopathic Method of Treatment.

It was, moreover, characteristic that all these patients expressed they knew something about the homeopathic method of treatment. P2 said: *'It was unexpected that I should delve into all nooks and crannies of myself. But as I am used to things happening elsewhere than where one thinks they are, I understand this method well. I understand quite well that the homeopath needs to ask about dreams and shock experiences; he tunes in on what kind of complex I have.'* P1 answered the question about how long the aggravation lasted, as follows: *'For some days, as it was the right pill I got. Once I did not get it (the right pill), and that one ought not to speak about, ought one.'* P5 said: *'But you can just as well experience that it (the homeopathic tablet) does not work, namely, that it is not the right one. And then you have to go over there again and speak with him. That is why I did not return to see him, because I was almost sure it was the correct pill he had given me.'*

Choice of Treatment

Four of the patients had seen a medical practicioner of the orthodox system of treatment regarding the trouble they presented with. One of these patients had no confidence in the treatment methods used in orthodox medicine. The other three patients were dissatisfied with the treatment they had received. P1 said: *'I had been up to 10mg Ritain per day seven to eight times in the beginning, and that is a lot. At that time I felt bad, because one actually gets very paranoid from it. I felt very bad'.*

The push effect away from the orthodox system appears to be stronger than the pull effect of homeopathy. P2 stated: *'I am very open to alternative methods of treatment, so I could have chosen many different treatment methods: acupuncture, biopathy, etc. I go to a chiropractor already, and also go to healing every now and then. I chose this homeopath because he was recommended by my friend'.*

Motivation

Three of the five interviewed patients stated that they had been especially motivated for something to happen with their problem at the time they consulted their homeopath. P2 said: *'I was about to go on a trip. I would probably also have come for treatment anyway, but I pulled myself together to do something at that time.'* The other two patients said they were probably motivated, but not especially more motivated at the time of starting homeopathic treatment than at any other time before, when they had tried other alternative therapies. P1 said: *'I have always been very interested in getting treated. This has probably not changed. I have always really wanted to do something about it'.*

Conclusions

As can be seen, the characteristics these patients had in common is a dissatisfaction with the treatment possibilities of the orthodox system. Several of the patients had been looking for an alternative method of treatment that would include the psychosomatic aspect.

These motives behind seeking alternative treatment have also been found in other, larger surveys (Hofmeister E., et al. 1994).

Moreover, another characteristic of these patients is that they expressed a readiness to talk about many aspects of their lives during the consultation, and that they were prepared to come for several consultations if needed. Furthermore, they had all contacted their homeopath again after the first consultation, either by telephone or in follow-up consultations.

That the patients already had an understanding of homeopathic treatment principles, is precisely the factor which homeopaths stress as being important for finding the right remedy, and thus achieving good results. The patients also expressed that they had been motivated for something to happen with their problem at the time they consulted the homeopath. However, it does not appear that the patients who had received alternative treatment previously were especially more motivated for treatment at the time they consulted the homeopath than the others.

Section 3: Questionnaire Evaluation.

In This Section the Following Questions Are Taken Up:

▸ What type of patient comes to classical homeopathy, according to sex, age and health problem
▸ What health changes had patients experienced after starting classical homeopathic treatment?
▸ Were the changes experienced by patients in agreement with the results and goals expected by the homeopaths?
▸ Was there any connection between the changes experienced by patients and factors the homeopaths considered might affect the results of treatment?

The answers are based on a survey made up of two parts. Part 1 consists of data collected from all patients who had started treatment with the seven selected homeopaths in the period from 01.02.94 to 01.02.95. In Part 2, data was collected from patients who, according to their homeopaths, had obtained a positive result from the treatment, and had started treatment or were still being treated during the period from 01.02.92 to 01.02.94. As Part 2 is primarily of interest to practising homeopaths, the results from this part will not be included in the tables and figures of this shortened version of the survey. The results of Part 2 will, however, be briefly described.

The design of the questionnaire employed was based on both the theories of classical homeopathy and the interviews made with the selected homeopaths and patients, and was thus designed to register any expected changes and some, which from experience might occur in connection with a homeopathic course of treatment, during a curative process.

The Patients Were Characterised by the Fact That:

▸ The treatment was carried out by a classical homeopath who at the start of the period had completed his training at the School for Classical Homeopathy (Skolen for Klassisk Homøopati) or was teaching at this school, the treatment being in accordance with the guidelines established by The Danish Association for Classical Homeopathy (DSKH).
▸ They had themselves chosen to be treated with classical homeopathy.
▸ They had chosen the homeopath personally.
▸ They had paid for the treatment themselves.
▸ Their treatment was given under normal treatment conditions and not for the purpose of this survey.

Reply Percentages

There was a total of 345 patients in the survey, 209 in Part 1, 136 in Part 2.

Part 1   69%:   Answered the returned questionnaire, a total of 144 patients.
         20%:   By telephone, by letter or by returning unanswered questionnaires expressed they did not wish to participate in the survey.
         11%:   Failed to respond.

Part2:   72%:   Answered and returned the questionnaire, a total of 98 patients.
         11%:   By telephone, by letter or by returning unanswered questionnaires expressed they did not wish to participate in the survey.
         17%:   Failed to respond.

The two tables below show how the patients questioned in Part 1 were distributed as regards the number of consultations and the length of treatment at the time of answering the questionnaire:

Number of consultations	% (N=144)
1	19
2	34
3	17
4	15
Between 5 and 9	13
More than 9	1
No response	1

Table 2. Number of consultations.

Length of treatment in years	% (N=144)
Up to $1/4$ year	4
($1/4$ - $1/2$)	19
($1/2$ –1)	61
(1-1$1/2$)	16
No response	0

Table 3. Length of treatment.

PATIENTS OF CLASSICAL HOMEOPATHY BY SEX, AGE AND HEALTH PROBLEM

Sex and Age Distribution of Patients of Classical Homeopathy

The survey showed a clear majority of female patients using classical homeopathy (72%).

As can be seen in figure 4, the greatest percentage (67%) of the patients were between the ages of 20 and 49 years, distributed in the following age groups: 20-29 years, 18%; 30-39 years, 28%; and 40-49 years, 21%. This pattern regarding sex and age was also found in other surveys of patients who consulted alternative therapy (Launsø, 1995).

Moreover, the same pattern was found in a Norwegian survey, which showed that 66% of the patients who consulted homeopaths were women and the most frequent age group was from 30 to 40 years old (Lærum, 1985).

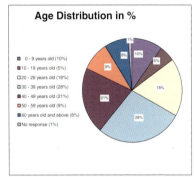

Age Distribution in %

- 0 - 9 years old (10%)
- 10 - 19 years old (5%)
- 20 - 29 years old (18%)
- 30 - 39 years old (28%)
- 40 - 49 years old (21%)
- 50 - 59 years old (9%)
- 60 years old and above (8%)
- No response (1%)

Figure 4. Age distribution for patients of classical homeopathy.

Conditions Patients Presented With

As can be seen in table 5, the survey showed that the majority (77%) of the patients presented with a physical problem as their chief complaint. The most frequent physical problems were pains (13%), skin problems (14%), infections (12%), and asthma/allergy (12%).
Moreover, half of the patients came with other problems of which 50% were psychological.
In contrast, a Norwegian survey showed that the most frequent maladies presented for homeopathic treatment were muscle and skeletal problems (about 15%), respiratory illnesses (about 10%), gastrointestinal problems (about 10%) and psychological problems (about 10%) (Lærum, 1985).

Health Problem	% (N=144)
Allergy	8
Asthma	4
Pains	13
Skin Problems	14
Infections	12
Gastrointestinal Problems	6
Heart and Circulatory Problems	2
Various Physical Problems	19
Anxiety	3
Depression	4
Various Psychological Problems	16

Table 5. The chief complaint patients presented with for homeopathic treatment.

Duration of Problem in Years	% (N=144)
0 - $1/2$	21
$1/2$ - 1	12
1 - 3	17
3 - 5	9
More than 5	37
No Response	5

Table 6. The approximate length of time patients had suffered from their chief complaint at the time of starting homeopathic treatment .

As can be seen in table 6, the majority of the patients had suffered from their chief complaint for less than one year (33%), or more than five years (37%) at the time they came to the homeopath.

CHANGES EXPERIENCED BY PATIENTS AFTER STARTING HOMEOPATHIC TREATMENT

As shown in figure 7, the survey showed that 73% of the patients experienced a change with respect to the chief complaint they presented with. Eighteen percent stated that the problem was fully gone and 38% stated that the problem was not totally gone, but much improved. Seventeen percent said that the problem was only a little better. That there may be a case of 'central regression' can naturally not be excluded, because of the retrospective design. The phenomenon of 'central regression' refers to the assumption that patients who have had long-term symptoms tend to seek treatment during periods when the symptoms are worse. Any improvement may therefore not be ascribed to the treatment alone. However, it is in this regard important that the results experienced by the patients were not registered right after one treatment. The evaluation of the patients reflects a longer time period, and in most cases a longer course of treatment. Moreover, a third of the patients had previously received orthodox medical treatment, which did not help them. But, it is quite clear that future surveys should be done that will be capable of taking the phenomenon of 'central regression' into account.

Results in %

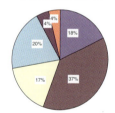

■ The problem is completely gone (18%).
■ The problem is much better, but not completely gone (38%).
□ The problem is only a little better (17%).
▨ No change (20%).
■ The problem is worse (4%).
□ Don't know yet (4%).
■ No response (0%).

Figure 7. The results patients experienced with their chief complaint as regards intensity and/or frequency after starting homeopathic treatment.

Twenty percent stated that they had not experienced any change with respect to the most important problem; 41% that they didn't know whether any change had occurred, as they normally would not have had the problem in the period when they answered the questionnaire. Four percent stated that the problem had become worse.

In all of the established disease categories an improvement had been experienced by some patients.

The fact that about 70% of the patients experienced an improvement also showed up in the reduction of medicines taken, (table 8).

Use of medicines		% (N=144)
Before homeopathic treatment	After homeopathic treatment	
No (60%)	No	59
	Yes	1
Yes (34%)	No	13
	Uses less medicine	11
	No change	7
	Does not know yet	1
	Uses more medicine	2
No reply		5

Table 8. Patient distribution with respect to the use of medicines for the chief complaint before and after starting homeopathic treatment. (By medicine is meant any medicine requiring a prescription, or any medicine that may be bought at a pharmacy to be used for a health problem.).

Of the 34% of patients who used medicines for their chief complaint before starting with homeopathic treatment, 38% said they no longer used any medicines for their problem, and 32% said they used less medicine.
Moreover, the survey showed that 56% of the patients no longer thought about, or thought less about their chief complaint in relation to before starting homeopathic treatment.
This was inquired about, since in the evaluation of the course of treatment homeopaths consider it important to know whether patients have attained increased freedom with respect to being mentally distracted by their problem, and not only whether an improvement of the problem itself has occured.

That 73% of the patients experienced an improvement with their chief complaint was also seen in another survey made in 1991 of patient results from alternative treatment (Launsø, 1995).

However, the present survey showed that only 18% experienced that the problem was wholly gone, while the survey referred to above showed that 33% experienced that the problem was wholly gone.

This difference might be attributed to the fact that different reply categories were used, or that the survey had a different design, among other things, with respect to the length of the treatment period. Or it might be due to the fact that classical homeopathic treatment, in comparison with other alternative treatment types, in general, has a lower cure percentage of the chief complaint presented. The reason for this may be that homeopaths are aware of the concept of symptom suppression, which for them is more important to avoid than, as a first priority, to remove the problem patients present with. The criteria for 'cured' are therefore different. Further investigations should be made to shed light on this question.
As mentioned above, a Norwegian survey showed that 91% of the patients who had consulted a homeopath reported they had experienced the disappearance of their problem, or had improved. A Swedish survey showed that about 75% of the patients had experienced an improvement, or experienced the disappearance of their problem.

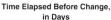

Time Elapsed Before Change, in Days

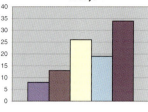

■ 1 day (8%)

■ 2 - 7 days (13%)

☐ 8 - 30 days (26%)

■ > 30 days (19%)

■ No change or response (34%)

Figure 9. The approximate time that elapsed after the first remedy was given before the patients noted any change with respect to their chief complaint.

Reason for Improvement

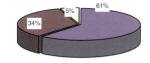

■ The homeopathic treatment (61%).

■ A combination of homeopathy and other things (34%).

☐ Other treatment (5%).

■ No response (0%).

Figure 10. The reason for improvement of the chief complaint, according to patients. Only those patients were included who experienced that their chief complaint had improved, 105 patients.

As can be seen in figure 9, 47% of the patients stated they had experienced a change with their problem within the first month after getting the first homeopathic remedy. Eight percent stated that something began to happen already within 24 hours.

Of the patients who had experienced that their chief complaint had improved, 61% said that they thought the reason for the change was the homeopathic treatment (see figure 10); 34% said that they believed it was a combination of the homeopathic treatment and other factors; and 5% said they believed the reason was something other than the homeopathic treatment. Evaluation of the patients might, in this case, be interesting in relation to the above-mentioned phenomenon of 'central regression'.

Changes Patients Experienced with Respect to Indicators Which Homeopaths Consider as Signs of Increased Emotional and Mental Freedom.

As is apparent in reviewing the experiences with classical homeopathic treatment of the interviewed patients and homeopaths, patients may experience a series of changes which are viewed by the homeopaths as changes in emotional and mental freedom.

In the questionnaire, the patients were asked to evaluate their own level with respect to this series of changes. They answered by checking off whole categories, assigning a rating from 0 to 10 for before and after homeopathic treatment. To this series of questions, the patients gave the interesting answers below. Beyond any changes experienced with the problem the patient presented with, the survey showed that after starting homeopathic treatment, *between 40-50%* of the patients experienced:

- That they had obtained more *self-confidence* (47%).
- That they had obtained more *joy in life* (48%).
- That they had obtained greater *energy reserve*s on a daily basis (50%).
- That they were more able to *accept themselves as they were* (43%).
- That they had become more *serene in their relations with other people* (43%).
- That their *spirits* had generally improved (48%)

Between 30-40% of the patients experienced the following:

- That they more often tried to *change things if dissatisfied with something in their daily life* (37%).
- That they more often *did something different than what they habitually would* (33%).
- That they more often *found new ways of solving problems* (35%).
- That there was a greater *agreement between who they were and who they expressed themselves to be* (35%).
- That they were less *worried in daily life* (37%).
- That they harboured less *hate and anger* (31%).

- That they less frequently felt *stressed* (35%).
- That they less frequently lacked *the courage to do the things they wanted to do* (33%).
- That their *sleep quality* had improved (36%).
- That they had become better at *expressing their feelings* (33%).

These changes are, as homeopaths understand it, expressions of increased mental and emotional freedom. Out of the 109 patients who answered all questions with respect to the above, 73% had experienced a change which was considered an expression of inner mental and emotional freedom. The table below gives all the information with respect to the above-mentioned emotional and mental changes.

Questions Regarding:	Positive Change %	No Change %	Negative Change %	No Reply %
Self-confidence	47	44	1	8
Joy in life	48	42	2	8
Changing things	37	53	1	10
Creating joy	26	60	2	12
Getting new ideas	33	55	2	10
New ways to solve problems	35	54	1	10
Energy	50	38	2	10
Self-acceptance	43	46	1	10
Serenity with others	43	45	0	12
Agreement with who one purports to be	35	52	1	13
Being worried	37	40	8	15
Jealousy and envy	17	66	4	13
Hate and anger	31	54	4	11
Stress	35	49	3	13
Courage	33	50	5	12
Being afraid and nervous	26	56	4	13
Mood	48	40	1	10
Sleep quality	36	56	1	7
Ability to express feelings	33	56	1	10

Table 11: The experiences of the patients as regards a number of emotional and mental conditions. N=I44.

Changes Patients Experienced with Respect to the Hierarchies of Vithoulkas
As mentioned in the section 'Classical Homeopathy', the Greek homeopath Vithoulkas developed a model, the cone model, which is used in the evaluation of whether the changes that take place in the course of treatment should be considered as positive or negative (suppression).
In the survey, patients were asked about every one of these hierarchies of the physical, emotional and mental planes. This was done partly to ascertain whether there were several changes taking place, and partly to evaluate the course of treatment on the basis of the homeopathic model.
Each reply category was checked off, assigning a rating from 0 to 10 for before and after homeopathic treatment.

As regards Vithoulkas' hierarchy of **emotional** problems, the survey showed (see table 12) that *between*

30-40% of the patients had experienced an improvement in problems with:
▸ Dissatisfaction (40%).
▸ Irritability (33%).
▸ Nervousness (35%).
▸ Depression (39%).
▸ Giving up, indifference, apathy (32%).

Between 10-30% experienced an improvement in problems with:
▸ Phobias (exaggerated fear) (23%).
▸ Anguish (21%).
▸ Suicidal depression (15%).

Emotional Problems	Positive Change %	No Change %	Negative Change %	No Reply %
Dissatisfaction	40	41	3	16
Irritability	33	47	6	15
Nervousness	35	47	4	14
Phobias, exaggerated fear	23	59	1	17
Anguish	21	60	2	17
Sadness	39	42	1	18
Giving up, indifference, apathy	32	50	1	17
Suicidal depression	15	68	1	16

Table 12. The experiences of patients as regards the emotional hierarchy developed by Vithoulkas. N=144.

With regard to Vithoulkas' hierarchy of **physical** problems, the survey showed (see table 13) that about 20% of the patients experienced improvement as regards:
▸ Skin problems (23%).
▸ Mucous membrane problems (19%).
▸ Problems with the liver and the gastrointestinal tract (18%).

About 10% experienced improvement as regards:
▸ Bone problems (8%).
▸ Problems with internal and external genitals (12%).
▸ Problems with kidneys and the urinary system (12%).
▸ Problems with lungs and the respiratory system (14%).

Physical Problems	Positive Change %	No Change %	Negative Change %	No Reply %
Skin Problems	23	63	4	10
Mucous membrane problems	19	66	3	13
Muscle problems	18	68	2	12
Bone problems	8	77	1	14
Problems with internal and external genitals	12	72	1	15
Problems with Kidneys and the urinary system	12	70	3	15
Problems with lungs and the respiratory system	14	72	2	12
Problems with the lymphatic system	4	80	0	16
Problems with the liver and gastrointestinal tract	26	57	3	15
Problems with endocrine glands	5	78	1	16
Problems with the heart and vascular system	4	83	0	14
Problems with the brain, spinal cord, neurones	3	81	0	15

Table 13: The experiences of patients as regards the physical problem hierarchy developed by Vithoulkas, N=144.

With respect to Vithoulkas' categorisation of **mental** problems the survey showed (see table 14) that between *20-30%* of the patients experienced an improvement regarding problems with:
▸ Absent-mindedness (23%).
▸ Forgetfulness (22%).
▸ Lack of concentration (26%).

Between 10-20% experienced an improvement in problems with:
▸ Dullness (lack of clarity) (15%).
▸ Lethargy (17%).
▸ Delusions (13%).
▸ Paranoid ideas (10%).
▸ Complete mental confusion (11%).

Mental/emotional problems	Positive Change %	No Change %	Negative Change %	No Reply %
Absent-mindedness	23	59	2	16
Forgetfulness	22	60	2	17
Lack of concentration	26	56	1	16
Dullness	15	66	2	17
Lethargy	17	65	1	17
Delusions	13	69	0	18
Paranoid ideas	10	71	1	18
Destructive delirium	3	80	0	17
Complete mental confusion	11	71	1	17

Table 14. The experiences of patients with the mental hierarchy developed by Vithoulkas, N=144.

Distribution of Patients with respect to Satisfaction with Results Achieved 'So Far' with Homeopathic Treatment

Forty-five percent of the patients stated that they were satisfied with the results they had achieved with the homeopathic treatment at the time of answering the questionnaire. Thirty-one percent stated that they were partially satisfied, and 20% were dissatisfied.

Satisfaction with Result Attained

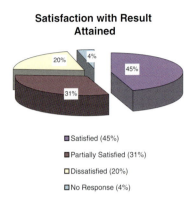

- ■ Satisfied (45%)
- ■ Partially Satisfied (31%)
- ☐ Dissatisfied (20%)
- ☐ No Response (4%)

Figure 15. Patient satisfaction with result attained.

Comparison with Part 2 of the Survey

Compared with Part 1, the patients of Part 2 of the survey included a slightly greater number of women (77%). Most of the patients (65%) were about 10 years older (30 to 58 years). No marked difference was seen with respect to the most frequent problems they sought treatment for.

In Part 2, the majority of patients had also had their chief complaint for less than one year (28%) or for more than 5 years (44%).

In Part 2, 90% of the patients experienced an improvement with their chief complaint. Thirty-three percent experienced that it was totally gone, 55% that it was not totally gone but much improved, and 2% that the problem was only a little better. Of the 36% who used medicine for the problem, 75% no longer used medicine (53%), or less medicine (22%) after homeopathic treatment.

Seventy-one percent no longer thought about (27%), or thought less about (43%) the problem. Fifty-nine percent of the patients of Part 2 had experienced a change with their problem within the first month, and 12% already within the first twenty-four hours.

Of the patients in Part 2 who had experienced an improvement with their problem, 71% said they believed the homeopathic treatment was responsible for the change, 25% said they thought it was a combination of the homeopathic treatment and other factors, and 1% thought it was something other than the homeopathic treatment.

For patients in Part 2, it was seen that with respect to the indicators considered by homeopaths as signs of increased mental and emotional freedom, it was largely with the same problems they most frequently experienced a positive change as for the patients of Part 1. Out of the 69 patients who had answered all survey questions, 86% had experienced a change indicating increased mental and emotional freedom. In Part 2, however, the percentage of most changes was about 30% higher than for Part 1. For example, 64% of the patients of Part 2 said that their spirits had become generally better, but only 48% of Part 1 said the same. The most frequent change in Part 2, as in Part 1, was that the patients had obtained greater reserves of energy in their daily life (67%).

The same pattern was seen with respect to emotional, physical and mental problems, namely that the problems most frequently changed in Part 2, were mostly the same as in Part 1. In Part 2, there was a difference compared with Part 1 in that the percentage of patients who had experienced improvement with most of their problems was between 15-60% higher.

In Part 2, 85% of the patients said that they were satisfied with the results achieved with homeopathic treatment at the time of answering the questionnaire. Twelve percent stated that they were partially satisfied, and 2% that they were dissatisfied.

The survey showed that the percentage of patients of Part 2 who had experienced positive changes, was larger than for the patients of Part 1. This was in agreement with expectations as the patients of Part 2 had been especially chosen as, from the point of view of the homeopaths concerned, they had obtained a positive result from the treatment.

WERE THE CHANGES EXPERIENCED BY THE PATIENTS IN AGREEMENT WITH THE RESULTS EXPECTED BY THE HOMEOPATHS AND THEIR GOALS WITH THE TREATMENT?

The Distribution of the Patients Based on the Answered Questionnaires.

Based on the answers the patients gave, the experienced changes were individually evaluated in relation to the expected results and goals of the homeopaths. The factors that went into this evaluation were:

Did the problem the patient sought treatment for improve, and was the patient now thinking less about it?
Was any consumption of medicines reduced?
Were there any positive changes with respect to the indicators of increased mental and emotional freedom?
Was the intensity of any other condition found in Vithoulkas' hierarchies reduced?
Was there a displacement in a positive direction, or was there a suppression?

Each questionnaire was evaluated and replies sorted into one of the following four categories:

1: Positive and Satisfactory
The changes experienced by the patients were in agreement with the results expected by the homeopaths from the treatment.

2: Positive, but Unsatisfactory
The changes experienced by the patient were in agreement with the results expected by the homeopaths from the treatment, but the changes were not great and/or the total condition of health was still unsatisfactory despite the positive changes.

3: No Effect
The patient did not experienced any change, or only some small changes.

4: Suppression
The changes experienced by the patient were considered a suppression.

Based on the homeopathic total picture evaluation of each questionnaire answered, the survey showed that 44% of the patients experienced changes that were in agreement with the results and goals expected by the homeopaths from the treatment, namely, positive and satisfactory as seen from the viewpoint of homeopathy. It will be interesting to learn more about his question in relation to the phenomenon of 'central regression'.

Changes Experienced

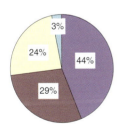

■ Positive and satisfactory (44%)
■ Positive, but unsatisfactory (29%)
□ No change (24%)
□ Suppression (3%)

Figure 16. Were the changes experienced by the patients in agreement with the results expected by the homeopaths?

Twenty-nine percent of the patients had experienced changes indicating that a curative process had been started, but the changes, at the time of answering the questionnaire, had not been marked, or the state of health after homeopathic treatment was still unsatisfactory despite positive changes.

Twenty-four percent had not experienced any of the expected changes or only a very few of them.

Three percent of the results of the patients indicated a suppression. This means that the total condition of health after homeopathic treatment was begun had deteriorated, either with respect to the intensity of different symptoms, or because of a displacement of the centre of gravity of the pathology in an undesirable direction, which in homeopathy is called a suppression.

Patient Distribution in Relation to Whether Past Problems Returned Briefly.

As described earlier, the homeopaths expected that, if the right remedy had been given, some patients would experience a brief return of past problems after the homeopathic treatment had begun. Among the patients of Part 1, 41% had experienced this, 45% of the patients of Part 2, as well. As for Part 1 and Part 2, 41% and 51% respectively of the patients who had experienced that 'old problems' returned briefly, had experienced them in reverse order to their original appearance.

Did Old Symptoms Return?

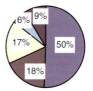

■ No (51%).

■ Yes, but not in reverse sequence (18%).

☐ Yes, in reverse sequence (17%).

☐ Yes - sequence not specified (6%).

■ No response (9%).

WAS THERE ANY CORRELATION BETWEEN THE PHYSICAL, EMOTIONAL AND MENTAL CHANGES PATIENTS EXPERIENCED?

The homeopathic understanding of human beings in relation to disease, health and cure is that the whole person improves after the right remedy has been given. Homeopaths expect, therefore, that beyond something happening with the chief complaint, there should also be an improvement in any other mental, emotional and physical health problems. Moreover, it is expected that the patient display indications of increased mental and emotional freedom.

As can be seen in the following text and tables, the survey showed, based on the patients' experiences, that there was a significant correlation:

1. Between improvement of the chief complaint and the indicators of increased mental and emotional freedom.

2. Between physical and emotional health changes.

3. Between physical and mental health changes.

4. Between emotional and mental health changes.

Moreover, by means of a logistic regression analysis for the patients of Part 1, there was found a positive correlation between improvement of the chief complaint and increased energy reserves in daily life.

These results agree with the homeopathic understanding of a curative process, and the expected results and goals of treatment.

1. Correlation between Improvement of the Chief Complaint and the Indicators of Increased Mental and Emotional Freedom.
In order to check for any statistical correlation in this regard, the changes experienced by the patients in relation to the indicators homeopaths consider as signs of increased mental and emotional freedom, were compared with the changes the patients experienced with their chief complaint.

The survey showed (table 18) that among the patients who had experienced an improvement with their chief complaint, 84% (66 out of 79) also had experienced positive changes with respect to the indicators homeopaths consider as signs of increased mental and emotional freedom. This applied to only 47% (14 out of 30) of the patients who did not experience an improvement with their chief complaint. Thus, a connection between improvement of the chief complaint and positive changes with respect to emotional and mental freedom was indicated.

Emotional and Mental Freedom	Chief Complaint		
	No Improvement	Improvement	Total
No Positive Change	16	13	29
Positive Change	14	66	80
Total	30	79	109

Table 18. Correlation between improvement of the chief complaint and the indicators homeopaths consider as signs of increased emotional and mental freedom. N=109, 35 patients were not included in this test.

A x^2 -test with Yates' correction applied showed that the observed differences could not assumed to be due to random factors alone, when tested at a 5% significance level.

The same pattern was found for Part 2, where Fisher's Exact test also showed that the observed differences could not be attributed to random influences alone, when testing at a 5% significance level.

Thus, there was seen a significant correlation, agreeing with the homeopaths' understanding of what happens when a curative process has been started.

2. Connection between Physical and Emotional Health Changes.

The survey also looked at whether there was any correlation between changes experienced on any of the three planes, the physical, the emotional and the mental, i.e. whether any tendency to a positive change on one plane would reflect on the other planes. Some readers will perhaps feel that the survey was testing for completely trivial correlations. Such testing ought, however, to be seen as checking the assumptions of homeopaths as regards results occurring during a course of treatment (see section 1).

With respect to any correlation between physical and emotional health changes experienced by the patients (table 19), the survey showed that among the patients who had experienced a total positive physical change, 76% (48 of the 63) had also experienced a total positive emotional change. This applied only to 20% (7 out of 20) of the patients who did not experience a total positive physical change. This would indicate a correlation between physical and emotional improvement.

Changes with Emotional Problems	Changes with Physical Problems		
	No Positive Change	Positive Change	Total
No Positive Change	28	15	43
Positive Change	7	48	55
Total	35	63	98

Table 19. Correlation between changes with physical and emotional problems. N=98, 46 patients were not included in this test.

A x^2-test with applied Yates' correction showed that the observed differences could not be assumed to be due to random factors alone, when testing at a 5% significance level. This, however, was not the case for Part 2.

3. Correlation between Physical and Mental Health Changes.

With respect to any correlation between the *physical and mental* health changes experienced by patients (table 20), the survey showed that among the patients who had experienced a total positive mental change, 75% (30 out of 40) had also experienced a total positive physical change. This applied only to

27

42% (25 out of 59) of the patients who did not experience a total positive mental change. Thus, it would indicate a correlation between physical and mental improvement.

Changes with Physical Problems	Changes with Mental Problems		
	No Positive Change	Positive Change	Total
No Positive Change	34	25	59
Positive Change	10	30	40
Total	44	55	99

Table 20. Correlation between mental and physical changes. N=99, 45 patients were not included in this test.

A X^2-test with applied Yates' correction showed that the observed differences could not be assumed to be due to random factors alone, when testing at a 5% significance level.

The same pattern was found for Part 2, where the X^2-test with Yates' correction also showed that the observed differences could not be attributed to random factor alone, when testing at a 5% significance level.

4. Correlation between Emotional and Mental Health Changes.

With respect to any correlation between *emotional* and *mental* health changes experienced by the patients (table 21), the survey showed that 27 of the 63 patients (43%) who had not experienced a total improvement with their mental problems, had experienced total positive changes with their emotional problems, compared with the 41 of the 43 patients (95%) who had experienced a total improvement with mental problems. Thus, a correlation between mental and emotional improvement was indicated.

Changes with Mental Problems	Changes with Emotional Problems		
	No Positive Change	Positive Change	Total
No Positive Change	36	27	63
Positive Change	2	41	43
Total	38	68	106

Table 21. Correlation between emotional and mental problems. N=106, 38 patients were not included in this test.

A X^2-test with applied Yates' correction showed that the observed differences could not be assumed to be due to random factors alone, when testing at a 5% significance level.

The same pattern was found for Part 2, where the X^2-test with Yates' correction also showed that the observed differences could not be attributed to random factor alone, when testing at a 5% significance level.

There was thus seen to be a statistical correlation supporting the homeopaths' experience that when a curative process had first been started, then the whole person would be affected physically, emotionally and mentally.

WAS THERE ANY CORRELATION BETWEEN THE CHANGES EXPERIENCED BY PATIENTS AND THE FACTORS THE HOMEOPATHS CONSIDERED MIGHT INFLUENCE THE RESULTS OF TREATMENT?

Homeopaths know from experience that a number of factors may influence the result of classical homeopathic treatment. The factors mentioned in the interviews were the following:

▶ The number of consultations.
▶ Whether the patient had had a person they could confide in before starting homeopathic treatment.
▶ Whether the patient within the five previous years had seen a psychologist or psychotherapist.
▶ Whether the patient had used allopathic medicines during treatment, especially cortisone.

Moreover, in the homeopathic literature it is emphasised that patients should avoid drinking coffee during the course of homeopathic treatment.

As regards the patients of Part 1, a significant correlation was found between the attainment of positive results and the use of prescription medicines during homeopathic treatment. Among the 101 patients who did not use prescription medicines during the homeopathic treatment, 79% experienced positive changes, compared with 53% of the 32 patients who had used prescription medicines during homeopathic treatment.
However, this result should be taken with a grain of salt, as no background variables were taken into account in the testing, and as no significant correlation was found in Part 2 of the survey in this regard.

The survey showed, though, that there was <u>no</u> significant correlation between the positive changes experienced by patients and:

▶ The number of consultations.
▶ Whether the patient had had a person they could confide in before starting homeopathic treatment.
▶ Whether the patient within the five previous years had seen a psychologist or psychotherapist
▶ Whether the patient had used allopathic medicines during treatment, especially cortisone.

That the survey showed <u>no</u> correlation between the number of consultations and positive changes was surprising, as the homeopaths considered it an important part of the treatment that they in follow-up consultations should have the possibility of evaluating whether or not a curative process had been set in motion, or whether another remedy should be given.
The reason for not finding such a correlation may be the variability from patient to patient of whether a homeopath can find the right remedy within a few consultations.

Moreover, for Part 1, one found by logistic regression analysis, after testing for different combinations of background variables, that there was a positive correlation between the importance of the case-taking conversation for the patient's understanding of himself and his life, and improvement of the chief complaint.

SUMMARY OF THE RESULTS OF THE SURVEY

Below follows a summary of the results of the survey as regards the questions formulated at the start.

What Is the Model of Health and Disease of Classical Homeopathy?

Classical homeopathic treatment is a method of treatment where the individual is assumed to have a life-maintaining and self-healing force, the vital force. The human being is considered to be an integrated whole of this force plus something physical, emotional and mental.
An individual's disease complex is considered to be a unique product of the morbific influences he is susceptible to, and the optimal way this person's vital force reacts when it is insufficient in relation to any morbific influences it is exposed to. In placing symptoms, there is an inbuilt prioritisation in the self-healing mechanism, which allocates symptoms where they will be the least limiting for the person's freedom and health.
It is this self-healing mechanism which is assumed to be stimulated in homeopathic therapy. That particular remedy is given to the sick person which, if given to a healthy person, would call forth the same symptoms

as those of the ill person.

In the homeopathic evaluation of how healthy a person is, one focuses on the person's physical, emotional and mental freedom. On the whole, a person with limited mental and/or emotional freedom, is considered to be more ill than a person with limited physical freedom.

How Great Is the Treatment Effort Needed in Homeopathy?

The survey drew the following picture of the treatment effort needed in classical homeopathy:

▸ An in-depth conversation with and observation of the individual patient.
▸ The right homeopathic remedy (simillimum) based on the homeopath's understanding of the individual patient's complex symptom pattern, an understanding obtained from the patient's statements and the homeopath's observation of him.
▸ Follow-up consultations (follow-ups) and evaluation of whether a curative process has been started, and thus whether the right homeopathic remedy (simillimum) has been given.
▸ Any needed re-evaluation of the patient's complex symptom picture and a possible new search for the right homeopathic remedy (simillimum).

What Are the Expected Results and Goals of Homeopathic Treatment?

The survey drew the following picture of the results and goals of homeopathic treatment.

When the self-healing mechanism has been stimulated by means of the right homeopathic remedy (simillimum), experience shows that this will lead to:

▸ A displacement of the freedom-limiting pathology according to a predictable pattern.
▸ Increased physical, emotional and mental freedom.
▸ Increased energy and reserves of energy.
▸ Improved health problems.
▸ Reduction of any consumption of medicines.
▸ The last disease symptom to arrive being removed first.

Moreover, homeopaths have observed that symptoms patients have had previously may return briefly, and that some patients experience an aggravation.

What Factors Do Homeopaths Believe May Influence the Results of Treatment?

Based on the survey, it was apparent that the homeopaths considered that the following conditions have or may have an influence on the effectiveness of treatment:

▸ The homeopath's ability to find the right remedy (simillimum).
▸ The patient's openness and honesty.
▸ Whether patients take hormone medicines, especially cortisone, during homeopathic treatment.
▸ Whether the patient has been to see a psychologist or psychotherapist.
▸ The patient's amount of vital force
▸ The number of symptoms.
▸ Whether the patient has had surgery for the problem presented.
▸ The number of consultations.

Who Are the Patients of Classical Homeopathy as Regards Sex, Age and Health Problem?

From the survey (**Part 1 and Part 2**), the following picture of the patients of classical homeopathy became apparent:

▸ The majority (more than 70%) of the patients were women.
▸ The patients were mainly between the ages of 20 and 49.
▸ The majority of the patients had had their chief complaint for less than one year, or more than five years at the time they consulted the homeopath.
▸ The most frequent problems the patients came with as the chief complaint were pains, skin problems, infections, asthma/allergy and psychological problems.

What Changes Did the Patients Experience after Starting with Classical Homeopathic Treatment?

From the survey for **Part 1,** the following picture of the changes experienced by patients after starting homeopathic treatment emerged:

▸ The majority (73%) experienced an improvement of the chief complaint they presented with.
▸ Eighteen percent of the patients experienced that the problem was completely gone.
▸ Thirty-eight percent of the patients experienced that the problem was not fully gone, but much better.
▸ Seventeen percent of the patients experienced that the problem was only slightly improved.
▸ Twenty-four percent of the patients did not experience any change.
▸ Four percent of the patients experienced that the problem was worse.
▸ The majority (70%) of the patients who used medicine for their chief complaint before the homeopathic treatment, no longer did so or used less medicine.
▸ More than half (56%) no longer thought about or thought less about their chief complaint compared to before the homeopathic treatment.
▸ About half (47%) experienced an improvement of their chief complaint within the first month after having received the first homeopathic remedy.
▸ Of the patients who experienced that their chief complaint had improved, more than half attributed (61%) this change to the homeopathic treatment alone, and 34% attributed it to a combination of the homeopathic treatment and something else.

From the survey for **Part 2,** the following picture of the changes experienced by patients after homeopathic treatment was begun emerged:

▸ A great majority (90%) experienced an improvement of the chief complaint they presented with.
▸ Thirty-three percent of the patients experienced that the problem was totally gone.
▸ Fifty-five percent of the patients experienced that the problem was not totally gone, but much better.
▸ Two percent of the patients experienced that the problem was only a bit better.
▸ Five percent of the patients did not experience any change.
▸ Two percent of the patients experienced that the problem was worse.
▸ The majority (75%) of the patients who used medicine for the chief complaint before the homeopathic treatment, no longer did so or used less medicine.
▸ The majority (71%) no longer thought about or thought less about their chief complaint compared with before the homeopathic treatment began.
▸ More than half (59%) had experienced a change in the chief complaint within the first month after having obtained the first homeopathic remedy.
▸ Of the patients who experienced that their chief complaint was better, the majority (71%) attributed this change to the homeopathic treatment alone, and 25% attributed it to a combination of the homeopathic treatment and something else.

Furthermore, from the survey (**Part 1**), the following picture of the changes patients most frequently experienced in a number of areas that homeopaths consider as signs of inner emotional and mental health became apparent:

▸ About **half** of the patients (47%) had obtained more self-confidence, 48% had obtained more joy in life, 48% had obtained a better sleep quality, 50% had obtained more energy and 48% had obtained generally improved spirits.
▸ More than **a third** (43%) accepted themselves more as who they were, 43% had become more serene in their relations with other people, 35% felt less often stressed, 37% felt less worried in their daily affairs, 37% tried more often to change things when there was something in their daily life they were dissatisfied with, 33% more often got ideas to do something different than what they would habitually do, and 33% had become better at giving vent to their feelings.

Moreover, the survey showed that there had been experience of improvement with a number of physical, emotional and mental problems, where the most frequent with respect to emotional problems were: dissatisfaction, irritability, nervousness, sadness and giving up (indifference, apathy). With respect to physical problems the most frequent were: skin problems, mucous membrane problems, and liver and gastrointestinal problems. With respect to mental problems, the most frequent were: absent-mindedness, forgetfulness, lack of concentration and lethargy.

The survey showed that with the patients of **Part 2**, on the whole, it was more or less the same changes that were most frequently noted. However, the frequency of most changes was about 30% higher than in **Part 1**.
In **Part 2**, about **two-thirds** (67%) had experienced getting more reserves of energy in their daily lives, which also was the most frequently experienced change (50%) in **Part 1.**

A little less than **half** (45%) of the **patients of Part 1** were satisfied with the results they had achieved with the homeopathic treatment at the time of answering the questionnaire, 31% were partially satisfied, and 20% were dissatisfied.

The majority (85%) of the patients of Part 2 were satisfied with the results they had achieved with the homeopathic treatment at the time of answering the questionnaire. Twelve percent were partially satisfied, and 2% were dissatisfied.

Was there any Correlation between the Changes Experienced by Patients and the Factors Homeopaths Considered Might Influence the Results of Treatment?
The survey showed that there was no significant correlation between the degree to which positive results had been experienced and:

▸   The number of consultations.
▸   Whether the patients had had anyone to confide in before the homeopathic treatment.
▸   Whether the patients within the past five years had seen a psychologist or psychotherapist.
▸   Whether or not the patients had drunk coffee during the homeopathic treatment.

For the patients of **Part 1,** a significant correlation was found between the degree of positive changes and the use of prescription medicines. Patients who did not use prescription medicines, more often experienced positive changes.

For the patients of **Part 1,** there was found by logistic regression analysis, testing with different combinations of background variables, a positive correlation between the importance of the conversation for a patient's understanding of himself and his life and improvement of the chief complaint.

Were the Changes Experienced by Patients in Agreement with the Results Expected by the Homeopaths and the Goals of the Treatment?
For patients in **Part 1,** by evaluation of the questionnaire as a whole, it was found that 44% of the changes experienced by the patients were in agreement with the results expected by the homeopaths and their goals with the treatment, and there was a positive and satisfactory result. Twenty-nine percent had experienced positive changes, but not entirely satisfactory changes. About a fourth (24%) had not experienced any of the expected changes or only a very few of them. Three percent of the changes experienced by patients indicated a symptom suppression.
With respect to whether problems patients had had earlier returned briefly after the homeopathic treatment started, 41% had experienced this, and 41% of these patients, i.e. about 17% of all **Part 1** patients had experienced that these problems returned in reverse order of their original appearance.

As for patients of Part 2, 55% of the changes experienced were in agreement with the changes expected by the homeopaths and their goals with the treatment, and there had been achieved a positive and satisfactory result. Forty percent had experienced positive but unsatisfactory changes. About 3% had not experienced any result. Three percent of the changes experienced by patients indicated a symptom suppression.
With respect to whether problems patients had had earlier returned briefly after the homeopathic treatment had started, 45% had experienced this. Fifty-one percent of these patients, i.e. about 23% of the total of **Part 2's** patients, had experienced that these problems had returned in reverse order of their original appearance.

On the basis of the experiences of the patients of **Part 1 and Part 2,** there was found a significant correlation between:

▸ Improvement with respect to the problems patients presented with and the indicators of greater mental and emotional health.
▸ Physical and emotional health changes (though not for Part 2).
▸ Physical and mental health changes.
▸ Emotional and mental health changes.

For **Part 1** patients there was found, by means of logistic regression analysis, a positive correlation between improvement of the chief complaint and greater reserves of energy in daily life.

CONCLUSION

The goal of this survey was to give an insight into the theoretical assumptions which homeopathic treatment is currently based on, the method of treatment itself and any results experienced by patients from homeopathic treatment. No similar survey has ever been made of classical homeopathic treatment in Denmark. It was not the goal of the survey to make statistical generalisations. For this a totally different survey design would be needed.

The results of the survey were, of course, limited by the survey design chosen and by the limited time a half year's thesis work provides. As was stressed in the report, the survey design did not preclude that any other conditions besides the classical homeopathic treatment might have played a role in the positive evaluation of results attained by the patients from the homeopathic treatment. However, in this connection, we must note that 61% of the patients who had improved attributed the reason to the homeopathic treatment. But, further research will be needed to uncover correlations between treatment and results. Here, among other things, a prospective research design will be needed, in which the results of treatment are monitored over several years. It would in such work be rewarding to combine such things as biochemical measurements, for example, with the patients' own evaluation of the results of treatment.

BIBLIOGRAPHY

Adamsen, L. et al. 1986; *Vejledning i evaluering*, AKF's forlag, Copenhagen.

Andersen H. 1990; *Videnskabsteori og metodelære*, Samfundslitteratur, Copenhagen.

Ballin, *Mennesket og mineraler*, referred to in Pedersen K. 1986; *Homøopatisk håndbog*, p.50, Borgen, Copenhagen.

Bernard & Stephenson, *Microdose Paradox: A New Bio-Physical Concept*, 1967, - referred to in Pedersen K. 1986; *Homøopatisk håndbog*, 1st.ed., p. 49, Borgen, Copenhagen.

Bohm D. 1986; *Helhed og den indfoldede orden*, ASK, Århus.

Boolsen, M. 1991; *Forskningsværktøj*, Copyright Gruppen KONTEKST, Næstved.

Boyd H. 1981; *Introduction to Homeopathic Medicine*, Beaconsfield Publishers Ltd, Beaconsfield, Bucks, England.

Braun A. 1980; *Homeoterapins metodik*, AB Arcanum, Gothenburg.

Brendstrup E. & Launsø L. 1995; *Hovedpine og zoneterapeutisk behandling*, Sundhedsstyrelsens Råd vedrørende alternativ behandling, Copenhagen.

Bruset S. & Tveiten D. 1991; *Homøopati - fortid eller del av fremtidens medisin?*, Tidsskr.Nor.Laegeforen. Dec 10; 111(30): 3692-4.

Bruset S. in the book edited by Launsø L:., Skjerbæk K., Tingstad A. 1995; *Livskraft og mennesker*, 1st.ed., Akademisk Forlag A/S, Århus.

Bryman A. & Cramer, D. 1994; *Quantitative Dataanalysis for Social Scientists*, Routledge, London.

Callian P., *The Mechanism of Homeopatic Remedies-Towards A Definitive Model*, J. Compl. Med., 1985; 1:35-56.

Christie V. M. 1991; *Den andre medisinen*, Universitetsforlaget, Oslo.

Clegg, F. 1993; *Simple Statistics*, 10th.ed.,Cambridge University Press, Cambridge.

Cramer D. 1994; *Introducing Statistics for Social Research*, Routledge London and New York. Delinick, Alexandra N. 1991; *Are Pathologocal Symptoms Self-Organization Phenomena?*

Dossey L. 1982; *Lægevidenskabens krise - Universet og menneskets sundhed: det banebrydende paradigme*, Borgen, Copenhagen.

European Commission, Brussels, July 1994, III/3701/91-EN, Draft 4, Working Party on "Control of Medicines and Inspections".

European Committee for Homeopathy, 1994; *Homeopathy in Europe*. Developing Standards For Professional Practice of Homeopathy in The European Union. European Committee for Homeopathy, Rotterdam.

Fog, J. 1994; *Med samtalen som udgangspunkt*, Akademisk Forlag, Copenhagen.

Foos L. & Rosenberg K. 1989; *Fra biomedicin til infomedicin*, Munksgaard, Copenhagen.

Gerber R. 1988; *Vibrational Medicine*, Bear & Company Santa Fe, New Mexico.

Hahnemann S. 1990; *Organon, Helbredelseskunstens værktøj, At turde vide*, Thaning og Appel, Kolding.

Hammond C. 1993; *Sådan bruges homøopati*, forlaget systime a/s, Herning.

Harisch G., Kretschmer M, 1991; *Jenseit vom Millegram*. Berlin: Springer-Verlag,1990. referred to in Bruseth S & Tveiten D; *Homøopati- fortid eller del av fremtidens medisin ?*, Tidsskr.Nor.Laegeforen. Dec 10; 111(30): 3692-4.

Hesthaven L. 1985; *Homøopati- En alternativ behandlingsform*, Naturmedicinsk Forlag, Helsinge.

Hofmeister E, Launsø L & Brendstrup E. 1994; *Centre for Integreret Medicin - alternativ behandling i udvikling*, Institut for Samfundsfarmaci, Copenhagen.

Holm-Nielsen, N. red. 1980; *Klinisk ordbog*, 12. ed., Høst og Søns Forlag, Copenhagen.

Homoeopathy in the United Kingdom, Profile, (ca. 1992).

Homoeopathy in Germany '92, Profil; 1992

Homoeopathy in Norway 1992, 1992.

Jensen, M. 1991; *Kvalitative metoder i anvendt samfundsforskning*, Socialforskningsinstituttet, Copenhagen.

Johannessen, H. 1994; *Komplekse kroppe - alternativ behandling i antropologisk perspektiv*, Akademisk Forlag, Copenhagen.

Kleinen J., Knipschild P., Riet G.t. 1991; *Clinical Trials of Homoeopathy*, British Medical Journal, 1991 Feb. 9; 302(6772): 316 - 23.

Køppe S. 1990; *Virkelighedens niveauer - De nye videnskaber og deres historie*, Gyldendal, Copenhagen.

Launsø, L & Rieper O. 1993; *Forskning om og med mennesker*, Nyt Nordisk Forlag Arnold Busck, Copenhagen (latest edition: 1997).

Launsø L. 1995; *Brug og brugererfarede virkninger af alternativ behandling - en sammenfatning*, Sundhedsstyrelsens Råd vedrørende alternativ behandling, Copenhagen.

Launsø, L. 1996; *Det alternative behandlingsområde. Brug og udvikling; rationalitet og paradigmer.* Akademisk Forlag, Copenhagen.

Linde K. et al.; *Are The Clinical Effects of Homoeopathy Placebo Effects ? A Meta-Analysis of Placebo-Controlled Trials.* The Lancet vol. 350 September 20, 1997

Lægemiddelkataloget 1992, Frederiksborggade 4, 1360 Copenhagen K.

Lærum, Borchgrevik og Wiens, 1985; Tidsskift for Norsk Lægeforening nr. 34-35-36.

Mehlbye, J., Rieper, O. & Togeby, M. 1993; *Håndbog i evaluering*, AKF Forlaget, Copenhagen.

Nørlund I. 1964; *Kybernetik og marxisme- menneskets nye muligheder*, Tiden.

Pedersen P.A. 1972; *Eksperimentel påvisning af virkninger af potenserede substanser*, 14. Oct. 1972, nr. 42, Farmaceutisk Tidende, Dansk Farmaceutforening.

Pedersen K. 1986; *Homøopatisk håndbog.*, 1st.ed., Borgen, Copenhagen.

Prigogine I. & Stengers I. 1984; *Den nye pagt mellem mennesket og universet- Nye veje i naturvidenskaberne*, Forlaget ASK, Århus.

Profile of Homeopathy in Denmark, Dansk Selskab for Klassisk Homøopati, Frederiksværk, 1995.

Sankaran R. 1993; *The Spirit of Homeopathy*, reprint 2. ed., Homeopathic Medical Publishers, Bombay, India.

Schjelderup V. 1991; *Helbredelsens grunde - Alternativ medicin i nyt videnskabeligt lys*, Munksgaard, Copenhagen.

Sundhedsministeriets Bekendtgørelse nr. 632 af 5. juli 1994.

Vithoulkas G. 1991; *A New Model of Health and Disease*, North Atlantic Books, Health and Habitat, California.

Vithoulkas G. 1993; *The Essence of Materia Medica*, B. Jain Publishers (P) Ltd., New Delhi, Reprint Edition.

Vithoulkas G. 1992; *The Science of Homeopathy*, B. Jain Publishers Pvt. Ltd., New Delhi, Reprint Edition.

Walach, H 1992; *Wissenschaftliche Homöopathische Arzneimittelprüfung. Doppelblinde crossover-Studie einer homöopatischen Hochpotenz gegen Placebo*, Haug, Heidelberg.

Winther, J. 1982; *Undersøgelsesmetodik og rapportskrivning*, 6. oplag, Socialpædagogisk Bibliotek, Munksgaard/Uddannelsesforlaget, Copenhagen.